450

D1764744

APPLIED IRIDOLOGY

Volume One

by

Harri Wolf

First Edition 1979

ISBN 0-9602636-0-8

Published by:

National Iridology Research Association
P. O. Box 3950
San Diego, California 92103
and
Wolfoxx Press
1768 West Arbor Drive
San Diego, California 92103

Printed in United States

Credits

Art Director: M. Suzi Feehery
Illustrators: Barbara Moody
Linda Kramer
Photos: Jim Coit
Color Photos: Harri Wolf
Well Being Magazine
Cover: M. Suzi Feehery
Printed By: Interim Printing & Mailing Co.

DEDICATION

To Kopavi

Whose uninhibited joy, and
unconditioned love are sources
of inspiration. We have much
to learn from the children.

ACKNOWLEDGEMENTS

There isn't enough space on these pages to detail the wonderful support, assistance, and encouragement I have received during the past four years of work and study. I would like to express my deepest love and profound gratitude to everyone who helped. Special thanks for continued support to:

Suzi
John "Jace" Schmitz
Jeff Freiheit
James Vahjen
Dr. H. Sunday Meyers, D.C.
Dr. Bernard Jensen, D.C., N.D.
Barbara Salat
David Copperfield
Dennis M. Warren, Esq.
Sanford Troy, Esq.
Mom and Dad, brother Jeff
Larry Baker
Rik Foxx

Forward

Throughout history, humankind has searched for effective ways of diagnosing and treating disease. In every school of thought, from herbal medicine to modern surgery, the search for more effective means has continued. Medical progress during this century has been phenomenal. Yet even though we have eradicated smallpox, can sustain life indefinitely by the use of sophisticated equipment, and are even beginning to understand the secrets of our own genetic makeup, health is still an elusive dream for much of humanity.

Recently much attention has been given to preventive medicine: the concept of building-up health rather than waiting for disease to strike. As a nation, our concern for better nutrition, more exercise, and the control of manmade toxins in our environment has already begun to show results in preventing life-threatening diseases.

The diagnostic tools of the physician are severely limited in regards to discovering the state of a client's health. Subtle changes deep within the body may elude both the client and the physician until a painful condition develops. Accurate evaluation of the state of the clients' health is proving more and more useful to professionals as their clients become more interested in preventive care. Not only medical doctors but midwives, nutritionists, chiropractors, naturopaths, and other health professionals are finding that iridology helps them understand the total picture of their client's health and provides a valuable cross-check for other forms of health evaluation.

This book is intended to lay a groundwork for those who wish to study iridology. Although iridology cannot be learned from any book, the understanding of what one will see in the iris can be. Many popular articles, classes and lectures have been given on the practice of iridology. Unfortunately, many of them tend to give the impression that one can grasp this tool and use it effectively with a minimum of study. In my opinion, this attitude is not only misleading, but could prove dangerous.

With the hopes of providing high-level education for interested people in both lay and professional circles, I approached Harri Wolf several years ago about writing a series of iridology articles for Well-Being magazine. The resulting articles more than met my expectations. In response to numerous requests from students, professionals, and lay people, Harri felt the need to publish this expanded compilation of his articles, adding color photographs, revised material, and some new portions which seemed appropriate to a book format. It is my belief that this textbook will help lay a solid groundwork for your study of iridology.

Barbara Salat
Editor: Well Being Magazine

CONTENTS

LIST OF ILLUSTRATIONS

Page

2

PREFACE

In my work I have encountered many sincere, health-oriented individuals who expressed a desire to learn all there is to know about iridology. To those people I say, "Iridology is a life-time study. Our bodies are very complex, many processes and patterns are not yet recognized and understood."

This book is compiled for the sole purpose of providing simple, clear definitions and illustrations as a supplementary work to the textbooks available on the subject. It should be regarded as a preparatory teaching to the impending flow of knowledge as this embryo develops. It will surely do so as research on the subject becomes more profound and extensive. Success is imminent. Truth is.

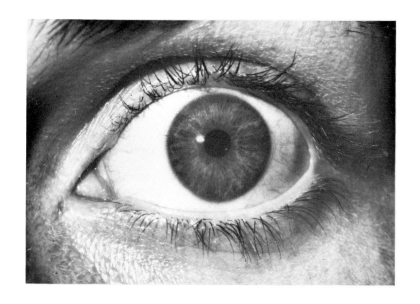

". . . In the immediate future, when our planetary life is somewhat calmer, the whole subject of vision and the registration by the eye of the inner worlds will receive an enormous impetus; and conditions—hitherto undreamed of—will be revealed. Man will enter into a new life and a higher era of understanding. The teachings concerning the iris of the eye is an indication of this. . ."

from *Esoteric Healing*

I
Introduction to Iridology

In every complex technology which mankind has devised, there is supplied a metering device, an instrument panel to engage a clear understanding of the internal mechanisms. Throughout the ages, the medical/scientific community has praised the human anatomy as being a precise, harmonious and wondrous phenomenon of nature. Now, wouldn't it seem logical that through some creative design, or evolutionary process (whatever the reader's preference), the human body would be equipped with a metering device functioning as a gauge in regard to the health of the individual?

Measure of Health Seen in the Eye

Each of us is, in fact, equipped with just such a miniature recording screen—the iris. Via the direct neural connection of the surface layers of the iris with the cervical ganglion of the sympathetic nervous system, impressions from all over the body are conveyed to the iris. Thus is established the neuro-optic reflex.

Iridology, as the study and analysis of the neuro-optic reflex is known, is the art/science revealing the pathological, structural and functional disturbances in the human body. To the trained and experienced practitioner, the iris reveals inherent characteristics of body tissue, the presence of acids, catarrh and anaemia potential. She or he can determine the acute, sub-acute, chronic or destructive stage of any affected organ through its corresponding sector in the iris. The conditions of the autonomic and cerebro-spinal nervous systems, in relationship to the organs, may be determined. Iris analysis reveals also the "hypo-" or "hyper-" functioning of the various glands of the endocrine system.

As a tool in preventative medicine, the iris can reveal the predisposition to certain disorders as well as some disease processes long before they reach the awareness threshold (often through pain). Iridology is still an embryonic science. Often, certain aspects are disputed by practitioners of the various schools. I feel that it is an invaluable tool to be used in conjunction with other diagnostic approaches whenever possible. I do not diagnose. I describe how disorders in a pre-supposedly healthy vital body are behaving. I do this by describing a number of phenomena and facts which constitute a total picture. To assist the health professional, I list the various expressions of the disturbed physiological functioning as portrayed in the iris. Then, he or she may choose to formulate a diagnosis.

In my view, the iris is a meter of constitutional totality. Let me explain. Disease is not an actual entity. It is a name given for classification purposes to the primary symptom manifestations and those manifestations of a departure from a state of equilibrium. No two individuals are alike in sickness

8

or in health. Though two people may be assigned the same disease classification, the patterns and processes that manifest the influence of the so-called disease are demonstrated by the iris to be highly individualistic.

Learning From Looking

I would like to share with the reader some of the great lessons taught to me by the iris.

First of all, the health and vitality of the gastro-intestinal system greatly affects the systemic equilibrium. The small intestines and the colon, through links in the autonomic nervous system and their roles in nutritive absorption, have a tremendous influence upon the other organs of the body.

I have also learned that suppression of acute elimination is one of the greatest dangers of modern medicine. Drugs often mask the illness, or worse, alter it in some fundamental way, pushing it deeper within the tissue of the body. This is often demonstrated in the iris by the diverging of fibers on the surface layers into arcs exposing deeper layers.

True, long-term healing can only come about with homeopathy and natural therapeutics. There are distinct signs that appear in the iris that demonstrate when a healing process is occurring. I consider it a blessing to be able to observe first-hand this process as it occurs—and I am always deeply affected by this phenomenon.

And finally, I have learned that health is not a state free from illness, and illness is not the disappearance of health.

Step One: Iris Density

As an introduction to those fundamentals of iridology that will be discussed in subsequent chapters, I have chosen

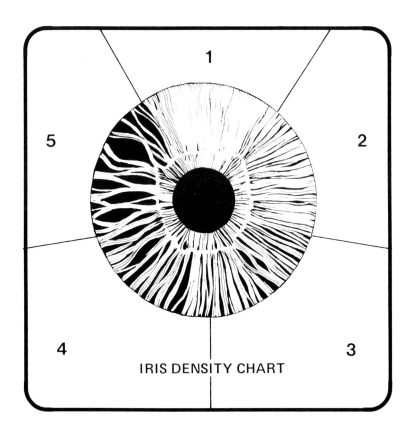

IRIS DENSITY CHART

the subject of *iris density*.

Look closely at an iris and you will see numerous fibers radiating from its inner edge, the *pupillary margin*, toward the periphery, the *iris root*. An iris whose *radial fibers* are arranged smoothly and lie close to one another is referred to as having fine density. An iris whose fibers are unevenly arranged, with openings or *crypts* between them, reveals a coarser density. *The measured iris density is reflective of the inherent strength and the recuperative powers of the individual.* This information is of utmost importance to the health practitioner who can evaluate it to pre-determine the intensity and the extent of the treatment.

In the accompanying diagram, the degree of density is represented by a grade of 1 to 5. An iris with fibers like those in section 1 suggests that its owner has a strong inherent constitution with excellent recuperative powers. At the other extreme, section 5 reveals a very weak constitution and a lesser ability to overcome disease.

Look at your own and other's eyes. It is not uncommon to find sections of loosely knit fibers in an otherwise dense iris. This suggests inherent weakness in the tissue reflex to the iris area involved. When toxicity prevails, these areas tend to be affected first and foremost.

Let me urge the student of iridology to pay greater attention and respect to the built-in durability of the human organism. We must learn to celebrate the absolute marvel to good health which is the true nature of most of us most of the time.

II
The Anatomy
of the Iris

The material in this chapter is the most complicated of the series. It will require careful study on the part of the interested and dedicated student. A bibliography is presented at the end of the book; it would be advantageous to locate and examine other reference material on this subject.

The *iris* is a thin, circular disc between the anterior and posterior chambers of the eyeball, forming a fragile and mobile diaphragm corresponding in function to the diaphragm of a camera. A round aperture, the *pupil*, is located near its center, slightly nasalward.

If you examine illustration 1, you will get a clear picture of the placement of the iris in relation to the surrounding structures.

A brief description of these structures is in order at this time. The globe of the eye consists of three concentric coverings enclosing transparent liquid media through which light must travel.

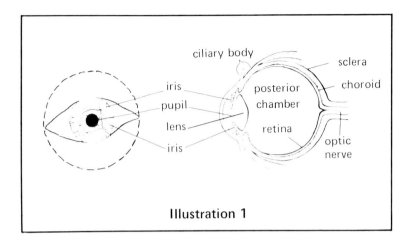

Illustration 1

1. **The outermost coat contains the sclera and the cornea.** The *sclera* is an opaque fibrous membrane, roughly spherical in shape, which serves to protect the inner parts of the eyeball from injury. It forms the principal part (94%) of the area of the outer coat. The *cornea* is a transparent continuation of the sclera which covers the frontal portion of the eye, enclosing the *anterior chamber*, which contains the fluid aqueous humor.

2. **The middle coat contains the choroid and ciliary bodies and the iris.** The *choroid* coat is a long, thin, pigmented tissue consisting mainly of blood vessels which nourish the outer retina. It provides a pathway for the vessels that supply the anterior eye. The *ciliary body* is a continuation of the *choroid* extending to the iris. Aside from channeling nutriment to the iris, it is responsible for production of the aqueous humor.

3. **The innermost coat contains the retina.** The *retina*, an extension of the *optic nerve*, forms the true receptive portion for visual expressions.

The adult iris consists from front to back of the following layers: (illustration 2)
- A. *Anterior endothelium*
- B. *Anterior border layer*
- C. *Stroma or Vascular layer*
- D. *Posterior membrane*
- E. *Posterior epithelium*

Description:

A. The *anterior endothelium* is a single layer of flattened cells. It is a continuation of the posterior surface of the cornea. Due to its microscopic nature, this layer will have little significance in our study of the iris.

B. The *anterior border layer* consists of intertwining processes of connective tissue and pigment cells. Depending on its density and pigmentation, this layer has a great deal to do with the color of the iris. In the blue iris, this layer is thin and has only a few pigment cells; in the brown iris, it is thick and densely pigmented.

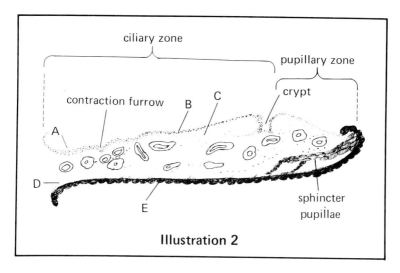

Illustration 2

The *anterior border layer* is deficient at the *crypts* and thinned at the *contraction furrows* (see illustration 3). This is very significant in iris analysis and will be discussed in subsequent chapters.

C. The *stroma* constitutes the bulk of the iris. In it are blood vessels running radially, giving rise to the streaks which can be seen on the anterior surface. These are enmeshed in connective tissue.

Illustration 3 shows how radial branches of the arteries and veins extend toward the *pupillary zone*, through the *ciliary zone* of the iris. The arteries form the incomplete *minor arterial circle* at the *collarette*, which henceforth we will refer to as· the *autonomic nerve wreath*. It should be noted that the course of these vessels is sinuous to allow for iris movement. The vessels become wavy as the pupil dilates and straighten out as the pupil constricts. Constriction of the pupil is caused by the *sphincter pupillae*, a muscle encircling the *pupillary margin* deep inside the stroma layer.

D. The *posterior membrane*, also known as the *dilator layer*, consists of a thin layer of plain muscle fiber. When it contracts, it draws the pupillary margin inward and this dilates the pupil.

E. The *posterior epithelium* consists of two layers of highly-pigmented cells. These line the back of the iris and curl around the pupillary margin, giving rise to the black fringe, or *pigment ruff*, which can be seen with the naked

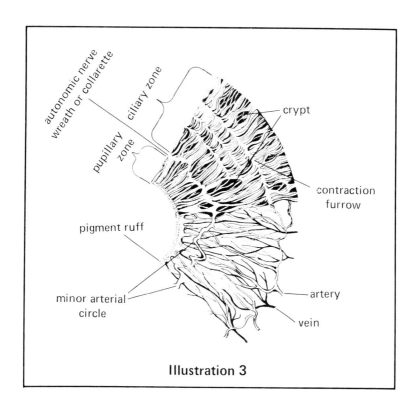

autonomic nerve
wreath or collarette

ciliary zone

pupillary
zone

crypt

contraction
furrow

pigment ruff

minor arterial
circle

artery

vein

Illustration 3

eye. This darkly-pigmented layer serves to prevent the penetration of light through the iris into the posterior chamber of the eyeball.

It will be necessary to review this material several times in order to become familiar with the structure of the iris. In subsequent chapters of this book, we will relate this information to what we see when we examine the iris.

III
Iris
Topography

We will present the subject of iris topography in two parts: I. Circular division; and II. Iris relief and iris chart development.

From a student's viewpoint, it is absolutely necessary to study and memorize the topographical divisions of the iris. This chapter contains a review of two widely-respected interpretations of the circular divisions and their meanings.

It is generally agreed that the iris can be divided into concentric rings or zones. Illustration 4 first appeared in Dr. Jensen's book *The Science and Practice of Iridology*. He shows a sevenfold circular division illustrating the zones in which various organs are placed. Thus, we find the stomach in zone 1, the intestines in zone 2 and so on. Please note that the line between zones 2 and 3 represents the collarette or autonomic nerve wreath.

A question that frequently arises concerns the placement of organs according to the zone chart as opposed to their placement in the diagnostic chart (see Chapter 4). There is no conflict here. If you superimpose a zone chart over a diagnostic chart, you can often pinpoint the precise location of signs. This can be a handy tool. For example, the fact that the lungs are placed in zone 4 does not mean they appear in zone 4 anywhere in the iris. It means that the lungs are to be found in zone 4 within the confines outlined by the diagnostic chart.

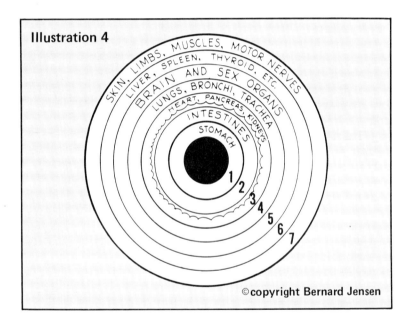

Illustration 4

©copyright Bernard Jensen

Another way of mapping the iris was presented by Theodore Kriege. According to Kriege's *The Fundamental Basis of Iris Diagnosis*, the iris divides into equal zones, three major or six minor (see illustration 5). The pupillary zone, or major zone 1, is subdivided into minor zones 1 and 2. Herein are contained the organs of food preparation and absorption.

20

The second major zone contains the organs of structure and support and "ultimate utilization, including detoxification and elimination."

Now, if you compare the accompanying illustrations, you may notice what seem to be a few discrepancies (for example, placement of blood and lymph). Remember, iridology is in its embryonic stage of development. Much research needs to be done. I am of the opinion that there are no precisely-defined borders. In my work, I have found that the importance of studying the circular divisions lies in discerning

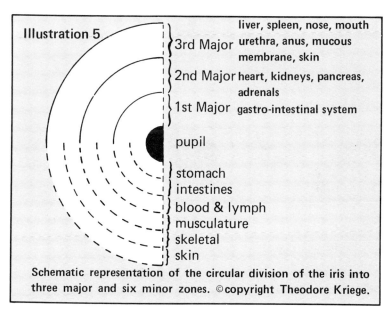

Illustration 5

3rd Major — liver, spleen, nose, mouth urethra, anus, mucous membrane, skin

2nd Major — heart, kidneys, pancreas, adrenals

1st Major — gastro-intestinal system

pupil

stomach
intestines
blood & lymph
musculature
skeletal
skin

Schematic representation of the circular division of the iris into three major and six minor zones. ©copyright Theodore Kriege.

the effect of a disturbance rather than its exact location. In addition, the *limits of each zone may be more or less expanded according to the cause which produces a sign.* Finally, in iris analysis, *each zone represents a function.*

I think the reader will understand what I mean upon reviewing the following explanation of the circular divisions (see illustration 6).

Illustration 6

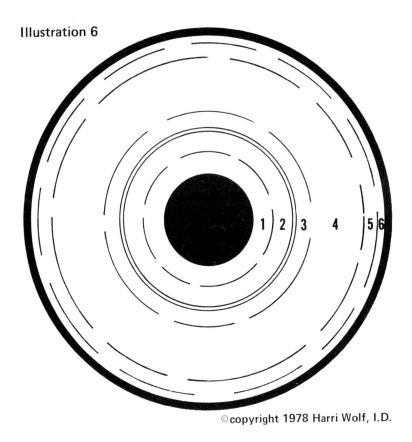

Pupillary zones 1 and 2 represent the nutritive gastro-intestinal system. These zones constitute the "hub" of the wheel.

Zone 3 includes the outer border of the autonomic nerve wreath. We know that any information we receive via signs in this zone is related to disturbances of the corresponding organs extending outward and inwards. I have found the root cause of many signs extending outward from this area to be found in the pupillary zone. Toxicity of the gastro-intestinal tract can spread via the lymph and circulatory systems, upsetting the sympathetic flow of energy and weakening the parts in the corresponding areas. Therefore, I view the function of this zone to be that of the *regulator of central circulation* (note: the heart is included in this zone) as well as the *harmonizer of the autonomic nervous system with the other organs.*

Zone 4 functions to expose the relationship between the organs represented here with other organs and systems, and with the body as a whole. All of the organs represented here have a relationship with the internal and external centers. By observing the nature of iris signs that have infiltrated into this zone, we can often determine ways to alleviate problems by applying therapy to related areas. For example, the infiltration of a skin zone sign into this zone in the areas of the lungs can suggest an overload of toxins in the skin area creating an encumbrance upon the lungs with subsequent stress.

Zone 5 corresponds to superficial circulation and to the lymph system in relation to the lymph flow in zone 3. We may find an expansion of this zone at times. Certain patterns of lymphatic disturbances are often seen extending beyond the borders of zone 5 inward to zone 4.

Zone 6 constitutes the skin. Its function is to demonstrate the complexity of the capillary circulatory system with regard to dermatological nourishment. Undernourishment and/or toxemia will damage the nerve fibers that activate the cellular system. Thus, perspiration and respiration of the skin is impeded resulting in diverse problems often involving other major organ areas.

When we consider the functions of the concentric divisions with regard to cause/effect analysis using wholistic concepts, and when we accept the fact that the outlines of the division are flexible, there appears to be no serious discrepancies between the interpretations discussed in this chapter. I would encourage the reader to gain a thorough understanding of all the systems mentioned in this chapter. Your experience will teach you the correct applications.

IV
More On Mapping the Iris

To continue our discussion of iris topography, we need to examine the significance of iris relief. The only publication I've seen that elaborates on this subject is *Iridodiagnosis* by V. L. Ferrandiz. In it is stated that one can categorize certain physical characteristics according to the relationship between the iris relief and the crystalline lens (see illustration 7). I have chosen to share with the reader those categories that I have been able to distinguish in my own work.

Illustration 7

1) Strong vital force; good equilibrium.

2) Fairly good resistance to disease. Previous disease has been resolved.

3) Glandular stress (possibly due to drugs) and irritated autonomic nervous system.

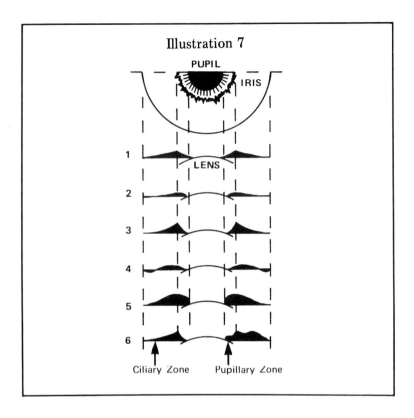

Illustration 7

PUPIL

IRIS

LENS

1

2

3

4

5

6

Ciliary Zone   Pupillary Zone

4) Reduced vitality; poor defenses.

5) Heart and circulatory problems including hypertension (high blood pressure).

6) Chronic disease; difficult to cure.

Continuing the Development of the Iris Chart

The focus of this chapter will be on the overall arrangement of the "map." Detailed discussions of field areas will be presented in subsequent articles.

To illustrate this discussion, I have selected the iridology chart developed by Dr. Bernard Jensen (see illustration).

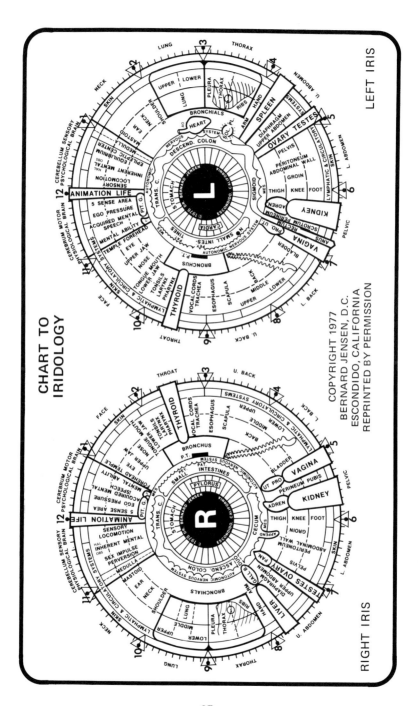

CHART TO
IRIDOLOGY

LEFT IRIS

RIGHT IRIS

I find it to contain the most reliable and consistent reference points of any of the charts I've seen. At some future time, I hope we can reprint and discuss some of the charts used around the world.

I hope to make the reader aware of the fact that the areas of the iris are not arbitrary signs, but that they have an authentic fundamental physiology that is related to every organ of the body.

We have previously observed that the area of the stomach is found around the pupil and that the area of the intestines circles that of the stomach. On the external border of the intestinal area, we find the *autonomic nerve wreath*, which, as its name indicates, is the reflection of the autonomic nervous system. All the involuntary organic functions and involuntary movements depend upon this system for "juice." From this wreath radiate the corresponding areas to the rest of the organs of the body, except the skin, whose area surrounds all the others. This is analogous to the fact that the skin surrounds the entire body. Since the stomach and intestines furnish the nutritive energy of the organism, it seems that their placement at the "hub of the wheel" corresponds harmoniously with the physiological condition of the organism.

I would like to demonstrate several examples of how the iris divisions are in harmony with locations of the various parts of the body.

Firstly, in the upper half of the iris lie all the organs of the head and neck, plus the heart and lungs. In the lower half of the iris lie all the organs that are situated between the neck and the feet.

Secondly, those areas located on the left side of the body appear only in the left iris, and vice versa. The spleen, for instance, is on the left side of the body, and is represented in

28

the left iris. The symmetrically placed organs, such as mouth, nose, genitalia and the paired organs such as the kidneys, ears and eyes, have corresponding areas in both irises.

Finally, let us not forget how the concentric divisions demonstrate the correspondence between the inner and outer portions of the body with the inner and outer zones of the iris. In addition, the internal parts of any one organ would be represented pupilward while the outer layers will always be found toward the periphery.

Anatomists have known for quite some time that the pupil does not lie directly in the center of the iris, but rather nasal-ward. (See Chapter 2.) Yet this chart and most others show the pupil to be centered. I have seen charts in which the pupil lies off-center. Although there is distortion of the areas, the differences are slight. In my work, I have had to deviate from fixed reference points many times anyway, just to account for individual differences. Let's not forget that the chart is only a guide. Only through practice and habitual study can the iridologist distinguish and compensate for the individuality of every pair of irises.

V
The Origins
of Iris Signs

A neuro-optic reflex study, or "iris analysis," should be conducted by someone who is trained and experienced in analyzing the visible changes that have occured within the iris structure of the eye. These alterations in color and fibrous texture are actual manifestations of underactivity or over-activity of the nervous impulses controlling the various functions of the anatomy. These manifestations, from which an unbalanced or diseased condition can be interpreted, are differentiated by their color and by their shape.

Herein, I will take into special account the origin of the white and dark signs which constitute the first consideration in the recognition of an unbalanced state. Some of these signs may suggest the accumulation of toxic metabolites. Other signs are a reflection of a particular stage of inflammation ranging from the acute or active (and sometimes painful) all the way to the destructive or final stage.

Let us first consider these simple rules:

White signs reflect over-stimulation, an acute process or hyperactive state of the nerves.

Dark signs mean diminished activity or insufficient stimulation; a progression toward an atrophic condition of the organ involved.

Fibers are made to appear white as the vascular layer of a given section of the iris becomes swollen in response to the congestion that occurs in the blood supply of any organ in an inflamed, hyperactive or congested state. This activity can cause the fibers to be raised toward the iris diagnostician and away from the underlying pigment layer of the iris. Thus is noted the lack of color and the white appearance. Please be aware that in the case of brown eyes, the observer won't see a white, but rather a lighter·shade of brown or even a yellowish coloration. In brown eyes we have to acknowledge the pigmentation in the anterior border layer. I would like to differentiate between three types of dark signs. The first is noted where the anterior border layer of the iris has receded to expose the vascular or stroma layer in response to an over-relaxed condition with a potential for tissue degeneration. A shade of grey indicates a sub-acute condition while an even darker shade signifies a chronic condition. These states are either inherited or brought about through suppression of an acute elimination process and subsequently an unresolved disease condition.

The second type of dark sign could appear as a result of toxic residue in the tissues (see illustration 9, A). Apparently as the waste deposits induce a degenerative process in an organ, the reflexive portion of the iris experiences a loss of fluid and a gradual destruction of connective tissue and vascular fibers. Very often, however, signs originally white can change to dirty white, grey, yellow or brown—often in the form of wisps or clouds. Such signs usually depict a sub-acute, or chronic long-term congestive state.

Black signs (Illustration 9, B) represent a degenerative state, or loss of tissue substance. These signs originate from the destruction of the stroma layer thus exposing the underlying pigment layer.

In the next chapter, I will review the origin and significance of the various shapes in which the white and dark signs will appear. With this, and the information contained in the previous chapters, we will be well-equipped to begin examining conditions of the various systems of the body as reflected in the iris.

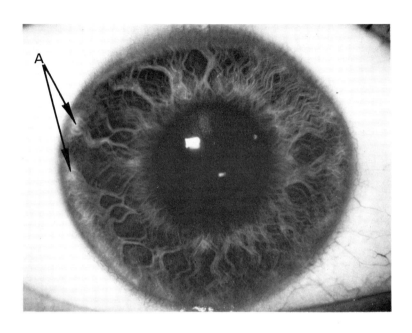

Illustration 8 Right Eye

A: White clouds in the lymph zone of the respiratory area.

What do you think is suggested by a darkened stomach zone?

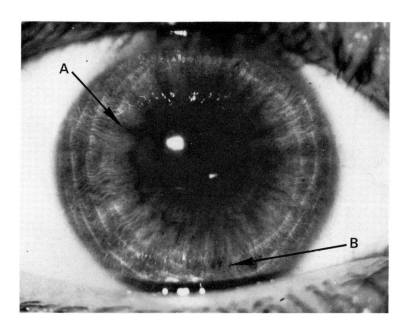

Illustration 9 Right Eye

A: Dark sign depicting toxic absorption

B: Note destructive signs in the kidney area

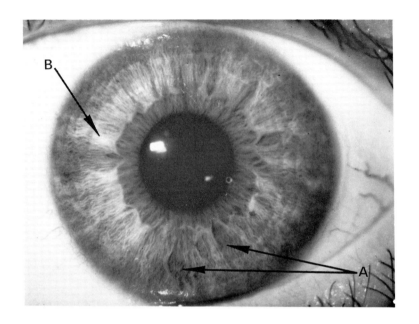

Illustration 10 Left Eye

A: Dark signs of the first type. These show conditions in the sub-acute stage. What organs are involved?

B: Shows an acute condition. When this photo was taken the patient had oppression in the chest with a very sore throat.

Do you see any chronic conditions here?

Where?

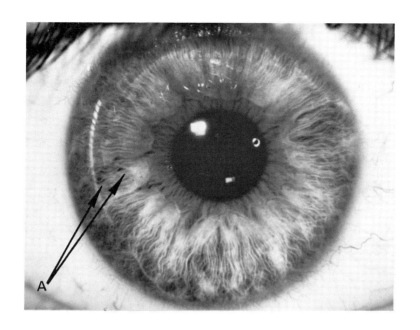

Illustration 11 Right Eye

A: Note destructive signs.

Note the overall white appearance of the central circulatory zone just outside the autonomic nerve wreath. This may indicate uric acid reabsorption which will alter body chemistry and undermine health.

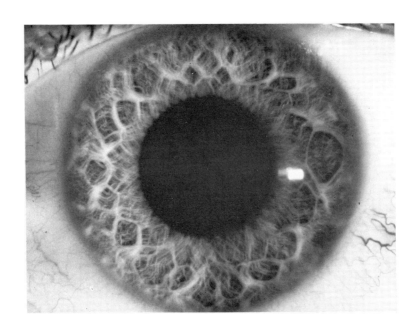

Illustration 11A — Left Eye

Apparent in the peripheral zone of this iris are the "cottonwool flakes," or white flocculations sometimes known as the "Lymphatic Rosary." People with these signs are predisposed to rheumatic disturbances, allergies, eczema, lymphatic and mucus congestion. I believe these to be genetically determined.

Color Iris
Photographs

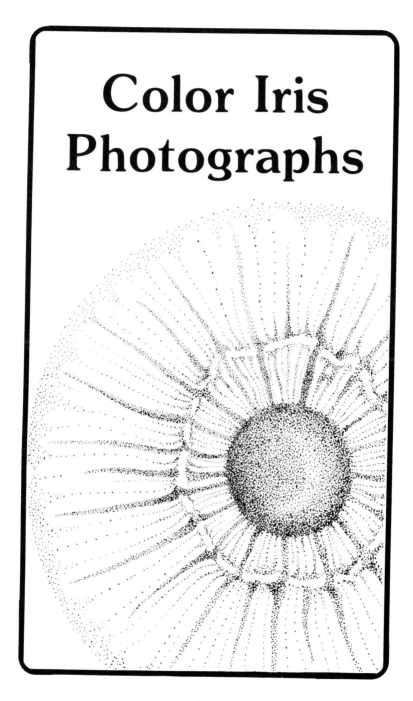

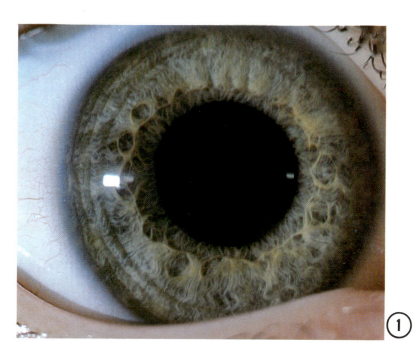

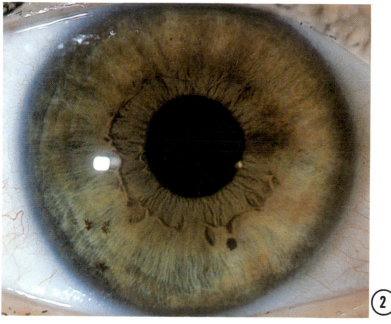

41

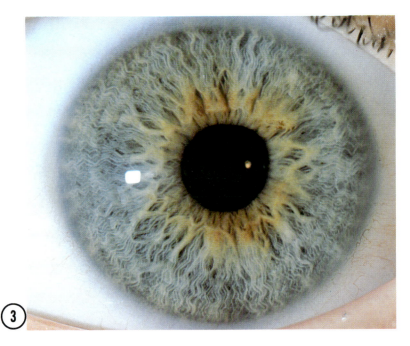

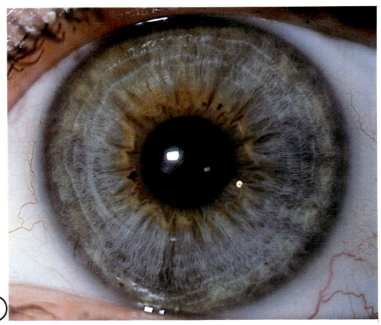

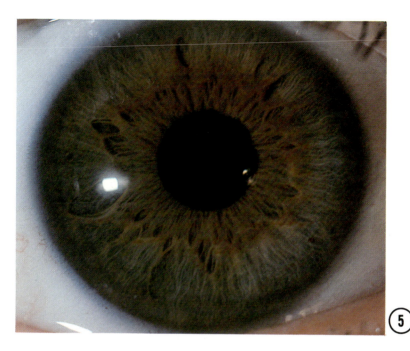

(5)

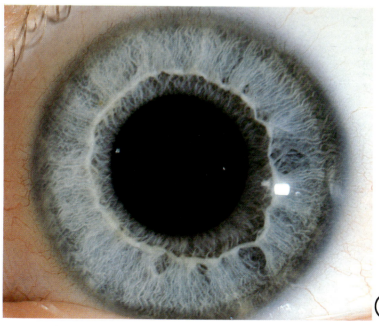

(6)

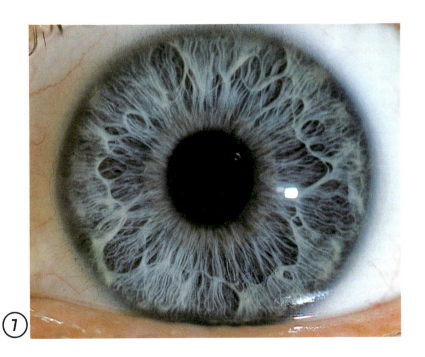

(7)

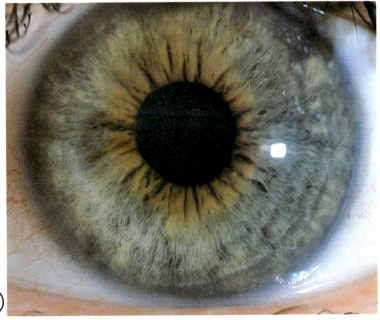

(8)

44

Discussion
of Irises

Note: It was not my intention to offer complete case studies at this time. Certain iris phenomena which will be discussed in subsequent volumes must be considered when undertaking a thorough evaluation. I chose only to discuss those concepts that have been advanced in this volume.

Figure 1. Right Eye

This slide was selected primarily to demonstrate a darkened and sunken nutritive zone suggesting diminished activity. Note also the deep contraction furrows indicating long-term inner tension.

Figure 2. Right Eye

Indentation of the superior Iris Wreath here suggests ptosis or dropping of the transverse colon with rather severe restriction of flow of fecal material.

Defect signs @ 48'-50' on the inside border of the Wreath suggest a destructive process. X-Rays revealed ulcers in the large intestine. Note the numerous contraction furrows suggesting much stress. Also observe the darkened skin zone. This often accompanies poor intestinal activity.

Figure 3. Right Eye

The sub-acute open lacuna @ 12' suggests latent inflammation in the pharynx region with toxic buildup and lowered resistance. This patient had numerous bouts with tonsillitis with pharmacological intervention.

Open lacuna @ 25' with clearly visible iris stroma suggests inherent prostate weakness. The white cloud and lightened radials just above this area suggest irritation in urinary bladder. This patient's father had prostate disturbances and patient reports frequent painful urination.

The closed lacuna @ 60' extending from the wreath indicates inherent weakness in the area often attributed to vitality. This sign may indicate tendency to fatigue.

Figure 4. Left Eye

Fibrous separation and darkening at 32'-33' indicates underactivity of the left kidney.

Irregularly shaped Iris Wreath, darkened nutritive zone and radii solaris indicate misconfiguration, stagnation and toxicity of the intestinal tract.

Yellowish clouds in peripheral zones indicate congestion and irritation of lymphatics and mucous membranes by noxious substances.

Note the darkened skin zone or "Scurf Rim."

Figure 5. Right Eye

Lacunae of varying sizes and depths are revealed in this

photo. The larger lacunae are surrounded by thickened borders. Look closely—do you see the fine knitting in these lacunae? What does this signify?

Figure 6. Left Eye

A white, raised and rounded Iris Wreath indicates an irritated and inherently weak Autonomic Nervous System.

The closed lacuna at 24' at the Wreath suggests inherent weakness of the left ovary. Note the fibrous separation from this lacuna to the periphery indicating hypofunctioning.

The small lacuna at 31'-32' at the Wreath indicates inherent weakness of the left adrenal gland.

This lady has a condition characterized by a loss of body hair, mostly on the scalp. Many physicians believe the etiology of this to be a combination of hereditary factors, nervous disorder and endocrine imbalance.

The iris does not label diseases. It illustrates the varying behaviors of the organs and systems of the body.

Figure 7. Left Eye

This type of iris, characterized by the numerous large lacunae and loose fibrous density, indicates a generalized inherent connective tissue weakness. Especially noticeable here is the loose structure of the intestinal zone along with the distention of the Iris Wreath. This indicates poor intestinal muscle tone and flaccidity.

The lightened and raised first zone indicates gastric hyperactivity.

47

Figure 8. Left Eye

Yellowish clouds in outer zones suggest noxious accumulations and congestion in lymphatic system.

Numerous Radii Solaris indicate stagnation of intestinal tract with subsequent systemic intoxication. Some noticeable terminal points for toxic materials are the Genito-urinary system, Parathyroid, and the cranial region.

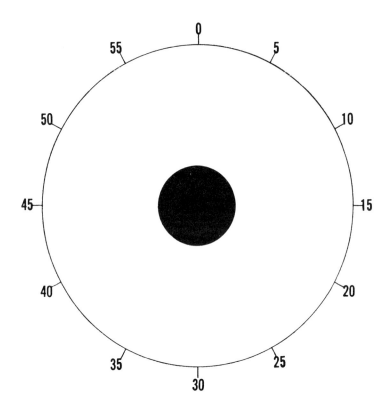

VI
More
Iris Signs

It has been said that "A picture is worth a thousand words." For this reason I have chosen to use photographs to further illustrate the nature of iris signs. In this and the next lesson we will pay special attention to the various forms of light and dark signs and their meanings.

Illustration 12. Left Eye

A: Wavy white line in the kidney area suggests an irritable condition, perhaps even painful.

Illustration 13. Right Eye

The white star surrounding the pupillary portion of the iris is noted in children and adults whose natural eliminative process is active with all systems working in harmony.

A: These white clouds—fibers enlarged and raised—are often associated with congestion of the lymphatic system. We call these flocculations or cotton-ball flakes. They are sometimes referred to as the *lymphatic rosary*. I have observed that many subjects with these signs in the lung regions of the iris confirm a history of ancestral tuberculosis. Yellowish flocculations reflect toxins which are acquired in a person's lifetime. The practitioner can follow a patient's progress during detoxification or fasting by observing for their disappearance.

Illustration 14. Left Eye

A: White sign denoting acute activity in the frontal portion of the head. White lines extending toward the periphery of the iris suggest an inflammation in the "running" stage. Here the sinuses are involved relative to intestinal irritability.

B: Dark sign suggesting destructive process in the medulla of the brain. The effects of this can be far-reaching because this portion of the brain controls many of the autonomic, involuntary functions of the body.

Illustration 15. Left Eye

Dark lines, known as *radii solaris*, indicate a channeling of toxic material from a stagnant intestinal tract. The iridologist must make note of the terminal points of these lines to accurately determine which organ areas are the dumping grounds for this waste. In this case the following organs are affected:

A: adrenal gland and kidney
B: prostate gland
C: thyroid gland
D: pituitary gland

Illustration 16. Left Eye

A: Radii solaris are caused by a separation and bending of the outer layers of the iris. Of course, the darker their appearance, the more long term or "chronic" the condition. Whenever by-products of intestinal putrefaction are distributed throughout the body, normal bodily function is disturbed and a stressful state arises.

B: Nerve rings, cramp rings, or contraction furrows are indicative of stress due to overtoxicity, acidity, mineral imbalance, emotional and environmental factors, overwork, hyperactivity or organic disturbances (lesions, tumors, etc.). They are caused by indentations of the iris fibers. These can appear dark or light depending upon the gravity of the condition. Interruptions in the rings can indicate the source of the irritation. Often the organ sector involved experiences cramping or rigidity.

Kriege, in *The Fundamental Basis of Iris Diagnosis*, states that these rings indicate circulatory disturbance in the tissue. This follows the logic that if there is tension or cramping in the tissue, the blood cannot circulate freely and toxic matter cannot be eliminated efficiently.

Illustration 17. Right Eye

A: Radii solaris penetrating the autonomic nerve wreath indicates a grave condition of putrefaction involving the stomach as well as the intestines. The central nerves will be disturbed along with the autonomic nerves. It is important to remember that whenever nerve rings are found in the presence of radii solaris, the iris suggests that elimination is poor and rejuvination will be a difficult task.

B: A darkened skin and circulatory zone, or *scurf rim*, indicates a reflux of toxic material from a poorly eliminating skin. Our largest single organ, the skin is one of the most important organs of excretion.

A wide and dark scurf rim protruding into any particular area suggests an overload of waste matter in that area. In this case the respiratory system is burdened by waste which a healthy skin would ordinarily process and eliminate. Therapy must be designed to assist the eliminative organs, primarily the skin.

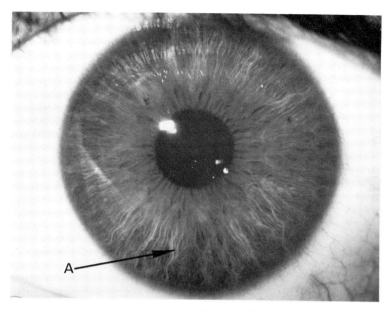

Illustration 12 Left Eye

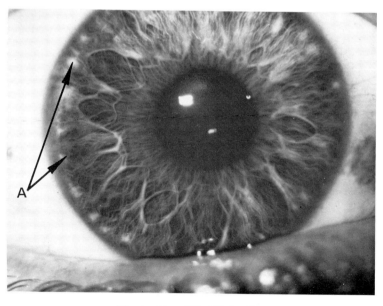

Illustration 13 Right Eye

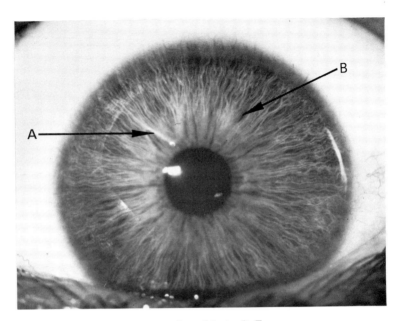

Illustration 14 Left Eye

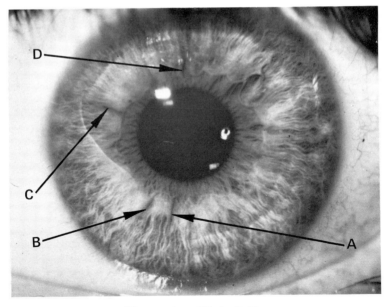

Illustration 15 Left Eye

54

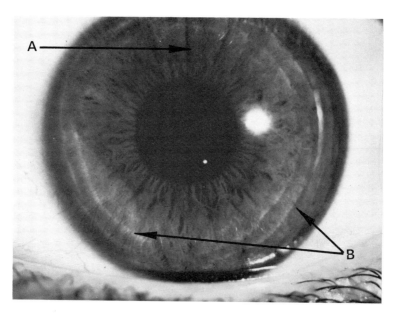

Illustration 16 Left Eye

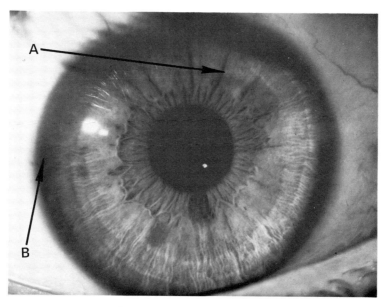

Illustration 17 Right Eye

VII
Change
As Seen In
The Iris

The following discussion of the signs and stages of inflammation will be the last of the technical data presented in this volume of the instructional series. The interpretation of these signs will be facilitated if the reader keeps in mind the various layers of the iris.

Known as an acute open *lacuna* (sometimes referred to as "lesion"), the sign in Illustration 18 indicates an active inflammation in the corresponding part of the body. Apparently swelling of the reflex area in the vascular, or stroma, layer of the iris raises the top layer. This can be distinguished by viewing the iris from an angle.

When this acute process runs its natural course, reconstruction takes place and the affected organ attains a healthier state. If, however, the acute inflammation is maltreated or suppressed, morbid matter is retained and vitality is lowered. The previously acute open lacuna now assumes a greyish appearance, indicating that destruction of the iris fibers has

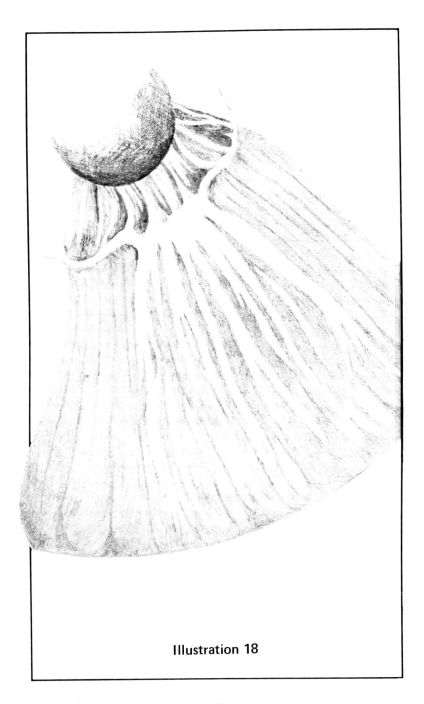

Illustration 18

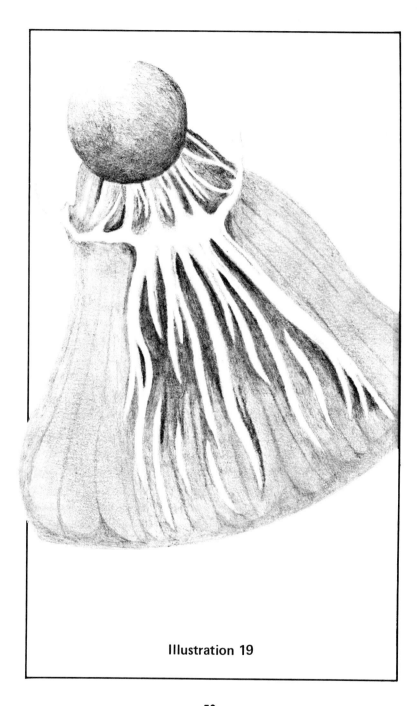

Illustration 19

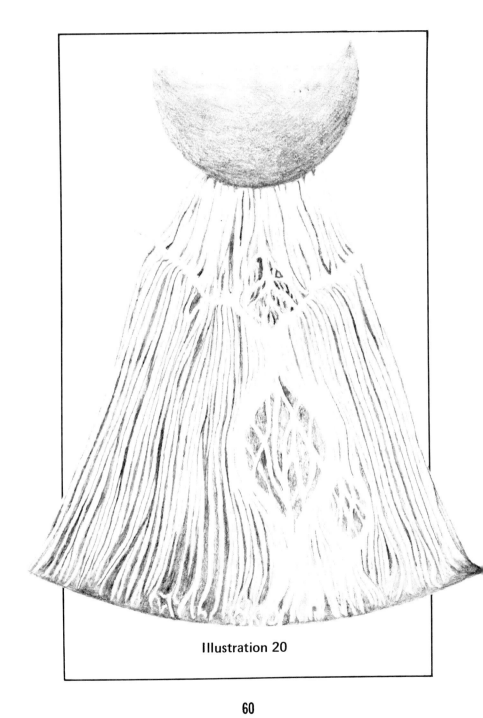

Illustration 20

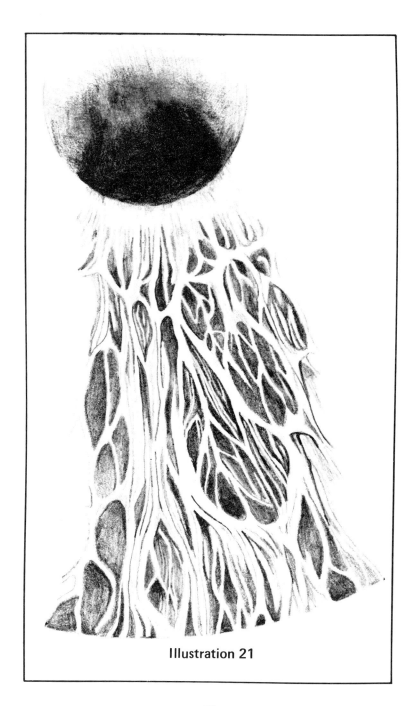

Illustration 21

commenced with subsequent decay in the organ that is represented. Under rational, natural therapy the sub-acute inflammation can be reverted back to the acute stage and ultimately eliminated. (See illus. 19.)

Often this second attempt at cleansing is suppressed and the sub-acute stage progresses toward a chronic condition. The grey lines and shadows in the iris become darker, indicating that the iris fibers are being destroyed or weakened. Separation takes place, revealing the lower segment layers. The chronic lacuna suggest that the body is depositing toxic waste in the tissue involved. Many times, due to weakening and damage to the nerve supply, loss of sensation ensues. I have observed that often the patient is unaware of the existing pathology, sometimes believing that he or she has been cured.

Closed lacunas are oval superficial structural formations in the iris stroma. They can be found especially in the fields of the lungs, the brain, the heart, the kidneys and the pancreas. Their diagnostic indication is a latent insufficiency of the organ, which sometimes only becomes clinically manifest with advancing age, trauma or infection.

The degree of iris stroma decay within the lacuna attests to the degree of weakness and often to the extent of morbid accumulations in the tissue. If nature succeeds in healing, the lacuna can become surrounded by and interwoven with white lines (illus. 20). These should not be confused with the honey-comb-like structural formations in the superior iris stroma (illus. 21). These suggest atrophy, inactivity, poor nutrition to the affected area or degeneration. Morbid material may be sealed off or encapsulated within the area involved.

Although it is not within the scope of this volume in the series to discuss the chromatic signs, I must say that these are some of the most important analytic signs of the iris. The variations in colors and shapes correspond to functional disturbances and metabolic changes. I believe that in most cases these signs are evident even before clinical manifestation. This testifies to the value of Iridology as a comprehensive tool in preventive medicine.

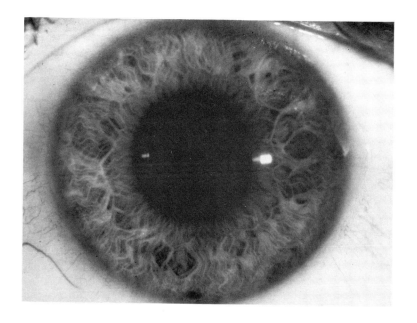

Illustration 22 — Left Eye

This photo demonstrates a closed lacuna containing destructive signs, or "defect signs" @ 30'-31'. Note also the wavy white radial adjacent to and bordering the lacuna under discussion indicating a state of irritation. This patient suffered from an inflammation of the bone (Femur) of the left leg.

VIII

The Examination

For this final chapter, I have completed a list of do's and don'ts. These are primarily directed at the beginner in the hope that he or she (whether a lay person or professional) can avoid the pitfalls on the path and be saved endless troubles.

Do's

1.) Keep an individual eye chart for each patient and put down markings you wish to remember. Devise your own "code" markings for the various systems as well as signs of disturbances. Be consistent with this code so that you will remember, at a glance, each individual case by simply looking at the chart.

2.) Be systematic on the procedure of the examination; this

will help you develop a smooth style, an aid in gaining the confidence of your patients.

3.) Breathe in a relaxed manner. Be sure your breath is not offensive. I often chew on a small piece of licorice root during the exams. This also serves to give me a more casual appearance and seems to make many clients feel at ease. Incidentally, you may wish to keep some handy for your patient. You can't do a good job if you must avoid getting close or if you stop breathing altogether.

4.) Allow the patient to rest the eyes at intervals by urging him or her to glance at a more distant object in the room for a while, or by closing the eyes. Do this yourself. I know when I become engrossed in my work I often stare for long periods and forget to blink. This can be tiring and stressful if you have a busy practice.

5.) Practice in your own life a faithful adherence to nature's laws. These are the truths revealed by our very fine art. The glow that will emanate from you will inspire others to explore these truths.

Don'ts

1.) Make no conclusive remarks about the patient's condition until the examination is completed. This may worry the patient. It has been said that a little knowledge is often worse than none.

2.) Never appear shocked or over concerned.

3.) Do not use medical terminology unless you are a licensed M.D. In other words, don't diagnose.

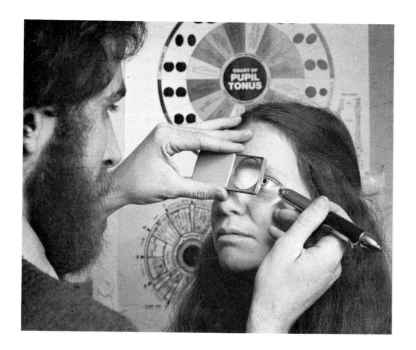

Equipment

Little equipment is actually needed for the exam. The vital necessities are a flashlight, a 3X magnifying glass, and comfortable chair for yourself and the patient. It is best to be seated so that you can look directly at the patient's eyes. A thorough examination may take from 30 minutes to one hour so it is important that you both be comfortable for the duration.

The camera is a very useful item in that iris photos are truly the most concise health records available. But as far as analysis goes, nothing can take the place of the direct eye-to-eye examination. Because of the iridologist's ability to move about and to view the iris from all angles, conditions may be discovered that can't be seen by the camera. The shadows and depths revealed by moving the light around tell a whole story in themselves.

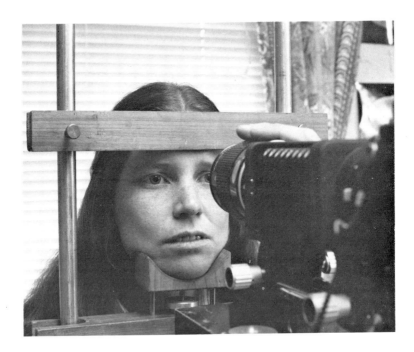

Method and Style

I often try to make my client feel that we, together, are arriving at the analysis of his or her state of well-being—that the iris is simply a tool I use to convey some of my insights into that person's condition. Though I may be able to interpret the whole picture from the iris, I usually allow the client to talk to me—to tell me when symptoms first appeared and how they manifested. This will often help me determine whether or not a condition is reflexive to an underlying disturbance elsewhere. Do not be afraid to ask for assistance. Be honest if you are in doubt or confused. What the patient may say in response will often dispel any confusion. Iridologists are not supermen. I consider every session a unique learning experience.

Keep in mind at all times that you are a health educator. Your role is to help others gain a thorough awareness of their bodies and an understanding of the fundamental interrelationships of its parts. You can only be effective if the patient trusts you. The patient must feel that in you he or she has at least one friend. Help that person to be candid with you by conveying an attitude of clarity, understanding and sympathy. God bless.

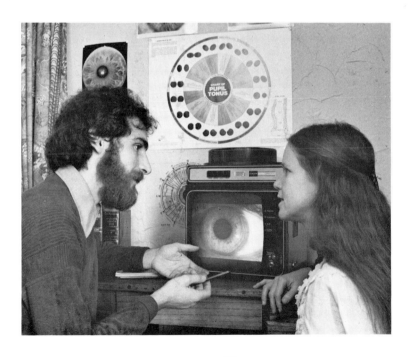

APPENDIX

Test Yourself

1-What does iris density measure?

2-Match up the iris layers   Posterior membrane=
    Stroma=   Anterior Endothelium=
    Anterior Border Layer=   Posterior Epithelium=

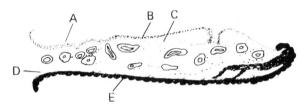

3-Which structure of the eye is responsible for channeling nutriment to the iris?

4-Which iris layer has a great deal to do with the color of the iris?

5-Which muscle of the iris causes pupil constriction? Where is the muscle found?

6-According to the author, what do the concentric zones represent?

7-Which zone serves as the regulator of central circulation?

8-Why study the skin zone?

9-What do white signs reflect?

10-What do black signs represent?

11-What does an acute open Lacunae suggest?

12-What do closed Lacunae suggest?

13-What do honeycomb-like signs suggest?

14-Which section of the Iris Density Chart
   suggests the strongest recuperative powers?

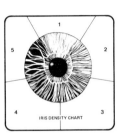

True or False

1-The iris forms the principle part of the area of the
  outer coat of the eye.

2-The pupil lies dead-center in the iris.

3-The radial streaks we view when examining an
  iris are nerve filaments.

4-According to the author, the study of the circular
  divisions can reveal the effects of a disturbance.

5-The boundaries of each zone are fixed.

6-Dark signs can be the result of a deficiency in the
  anterior border layer, exposing the vascular layer.

7-The chronic Lacuna suggests that the body is
  depositing toxic materials in the tissue involved.

Answers

1-Measured iris density is reflective of the inherent strength and the recuperative powers of the individual.

2-See Illustration 2, Chapter 2.

3-The ciliary body.

4-The anterior border layer.

5-The sphincter pupillae is found in the stroma layer of the iris.

6-The concentric zones represent functions.

7-Zone 3, including the outer border of the Autonomic Nerve Wreath.

8-We study this zone because the skin is an important organ of secretion.

9-Over-stimulation, acute process, hyper-active state of the nerves.

10-A degenerative state, loss of tissue substance.

11-An active inflammation in the corresponding body part.

12-Latent organ insufficiencies.

13-Atrophy, poor nutrition to the affected area;
or degeneration.

14-Section I.

True or False

1-False; the sclera . . .

2-False; nasalward . . .

3-False; blood vessels . . .

4-True.

5-False; may be expanded according to the cause which
produces a sign.

6-True.

7-True.

Iridology
Terms

Acute: *active, having a short and relatively severe course.*

Anterior: *situated toward the front.*

Anterior border layer: *a surface layer of the iris consisting of intertwining processes of connective tissue and pigment cells.*

Anterior Endothelium: *disputed outer-most layer said to primarily consist of flattened endothelial cells.*

Autonomic Nerve Wreath: *major iris landmark forming a concentric band around the pupillary zone and signifying the intestinal border and the autonomic nervous system.*

Catarrh: *inflammation of a mucous membrane.*

Cervical: *pertaining to the neck.*

Chronic: *long continued; may suggest some nerve damage.*

Ciliary zone: *section of the iris bordered by the autonomic nerve wreath and the iris root.*

Closed Lacuna: *an oval superficial structural formation created by the reconvergence of separated iris fibers.*

Collarette: *see Autonomic Nerve Wreath.*

Contraction Furrow: *see Nerve Ring.*

Constitution: *the make-up or functional habit of the body as determined by the genetic endowment of the individual and modified by environmental factors.*

Cornea: *transparent continuation of the sclera which covers the frontal portion of the eye.*

Cramp Ring: *see Nerve Ring.*

Flocculations: *light-colored flakey masses that are visible at the outer ciliary zone of the iris. Sometimes called "Lymphatic Rosary."*

Ganglion: *a collection of nerve cells that serves as a center of nervous influence.*

Hyper: *increased.*

Hypo: *decreased, diminished.*

Iridology: *as defined by Dorland's Medical Dictionary, it is "The study of the iris, particularly of its colors, markings, changes, etc., as associated with disease"; we define it as the art/science revealing the pathological, structural, and functional disturbances in the human body.*

Iris Density: *a measure of the proximity of adjacent iris fibers to determine recuperative powers.*

Iris Root: *outer edge of iris.*

Lacuna: *an oval shaped structural formation found in the superficial iris layers.*

Lesion sign: *see Lacuna.*

Lymphatic Rosary: *see Flocculations.*

Minor Arterial Circle: *an arterial formation forming a concentric ring around the pupillary zone of the iris. See "Autonomic Nerve Wreath."*

Nerve Ring: *circular grooves in the anterior layers of the iris which appear as arched segments. These are found in connection with stressful states, mineral deficiencies, tissue tension, and certain metabolic imbalances.*

Neuro-Optic Reflex Study: *Iridological examination; iris analysis.*

Open Lacuna: *a lacuna whose borders do not reconverge. This may suggest an active degenerative process.*

Posterior: *situated toward the rear.*

Posterior Epithelium: *A darkly pigmented iris layer which serves to prevent the penetration of light through the iris into the posterior chamber of the eye.*

Posterior Membrane: *the dilator layer of the iris consisting of a thin layer of plain muscle fiber.*

Pupillary Margin: *inner edge of iris.*

Pupillary Zone: *section of the iris bordered by the autonomic nerve wreath and the pupillary margin.*

Radii Solaris: *radiating furrows in the iris tissue wide at the base and tapered toward the iris root. Sometimes called "Sun Spokes."*

Retina: *the inner-most tunic of the eye. An expansion of the optic nerve, it forms the true receptor portion for visual expression.*

Sclera: *opaque fibrous membrane which serves to protect the inner eye from injury.*

Scurf Rim: *a darkened skin and circulatory zone indicating a reflux of toxic material from a poorly eliminating skin.*

Sphincter Pupillae: *a muscular band found in the stroma of the iris that contracts the pupil.*

Stroma: *the vascular layer, constituting the bulk of the iris.*

Sub-Acute: *somewhat acute; between acute and chronic; may demonstrate latencies.*

Wisp: *pale cloud appearing in the iris which may suggest inflammation.*

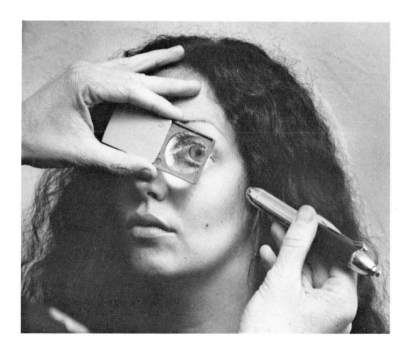

BIBLIOGRAPHY

Grundlagen der Iris Diagnostik: Deck, Josef,
  Ettlingen, Germany, 1965.
Iridodiagnosis: Ferrandiz, V.L., Ediciones Cedel,
  Barcelona, Spain, 1970.
Histology of the Human Eye: Hogan, Alvarado,
  Weddell, Sanders Company, Philadelphia, 1971.
Augendiagnostik: Jaroszyk, G., Medizin-Verlag
  E. Jaroszyk, Sols/Lahn, Germany, 1978.
Science and Practice of Iridology: Jensen, Bernard,
  D.C., Escondido, California, 1952.
Applied Anatomy of the Eye: Kestenbaum, Alfred,
  M.D., Grune & Stratton, Incorporated, New York,
  1963.
Fundamental Basis of Irisdiagnosis: Kriege, Theodore,
  L.N. Fowler Company, Limited, London, 1978.
Iridiagnosis and Other Diagnostic Methods: Lindlahr,
  Henry, M.D., Chicago, 1922.
Anatomy of the Eye and Orbit: Wolff, E., Second
  Edition, Philadelphia, 1940.

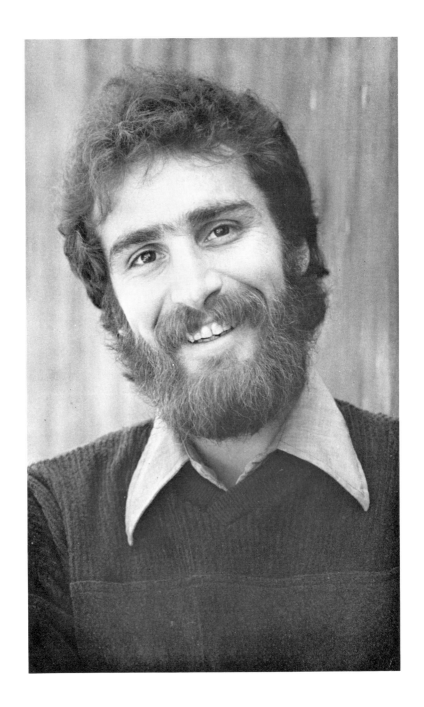

ABOUT THE AUTHOR

Harri Wolf has been practicing iridology in clinical settings for the past four and one half years. He is an adept lecturer and has taught elective seminars at colleges and other institutions around the United States. Harri is an iridologist and nutritional consultant for the Southland Iridology Associates and the Health Training Clinic in San Diego, California. A graduate of the State University of New York at Stony Brook, he is currently enrolled in a Ph.D program in Counseling Psychology with an emphasis on Health Education.

Harri Wolf is the founder and co-director of the National Iridology Research Association. He presently devotes much of his time to lecturing and presenting workshops throughout the United States and Canada.

ABOUT THE
"NATIONAL IRIDOLOGY RESEARCH ASSOCIATION"

The National Iridology Research Association (NIRA) was founded for the purpose of increasing and diffusing knowledge concerning the Art/Science of Iridology, providing a forum for the exchange of information and research regarding Iridology, and assisting the health practitioner in utilizing Iridology as a form of analysis, all with the goal of promoting better health care for the public.

In order to generate the funds necessary to carry out the principal objectives, the NIRA is engaged in the sale of Iridology supplies and educational materials, and the sponsorship of seminars and other programs.

Address all inquiries for information, brochures, and/or membership to:

National
Iridology
Research
Association

P.O. Box 3950
San Diego, CA 92103

Some of the products developed and distributed by the NIRA are:

1—INSTRUCTIONAL IRIS ANALYSIS
by Harri Wolf and James Vahjen
This package consists of high quality 35mm slides whose content highlight certain important phenomena based on iridological concepts. Case histories have been arranged to objectively correlate the iris signs with pertinent information regarding the patient. Case studies 1 - 20.

2—CAMERA STAND
An alternative to the more expensive and prohibitive iris-photo units available, this stand was designed for compatibility with most high quality SLR 35mm cameras with close-up attachments.

3—CHART OF PUPIL TONUS
by Harri Wolf
Compiled from decades of iridological investigations and personal experience, this beautiful full color diagram of pupil deformations with explanations of their meanings in relation to the body and the spine can be an invaluable tool for health practitioners and serious students of Iridology.